I0101250

A Simple Guide to Health and Success

Damon Moschetto

Absolute Author Publishing House
New Orleans, La

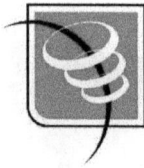

Absolute Author
Publishing House

A Simple Guide to Health and Success
Copyright © 2019
Damon Moschetto

Publisher: Absolute Author Publishing
Editor: Dr. Melissa Caudle
Cover Designer: Rebeccacovers

In-Publication-Catalogue-Data

Moschetto, Damon
A Simple Guide to Health and Success/Damon Moschetto
c. pm.
ISBN: 978-1-951028-14-5

1. Self-help   2. Health and Fitness   3. Body, Spirit, and Mind

TABLE OF CONTENTS

How to Use This Book

This is one of the most straightforward books you will ever read. At the same time, there is some gold in there, if you read with an open mind. Am I biased? Maybe, actually, yes, definitely.

These chapters are short and usually a rant on a particular health topic that you may or may not be doing, and if you're not, most likely should.

You could read this book cover to cover in maybe an hour. If it were me, I would read 1-2 chapters per day and marinate on it. Are you actually doing what is recommended in your life right now? If not, should you? And, if yes, then do it.

Some of this information presented, you already know, but it never hurts to hear it again. It may even be something you know but told in a different way that resonates better or worse (hopefully not worse).

If one of the chapters resonates with you, highlight and bookmark it. Come back to it when you need a little inspiration or kick in the butt.

Here is where I will insert my disclaimer. I am not very PC. I tell it like it is. If you are overly sensitive, this may not be for you. Here is your chance to bail but if you can handle a little tough love or simple truth, read on.

However, you use this book, I genuinely hope you find some value in it.

Introduction

If you are reading this, I am assuming it is because you want to improve some aspect of your health. It really doesn't matter where you are at in your health, the fact that you want to fix it speaks volumes. You understand that health is important, if not the most important thing you can focus on to improve your quality of life.

I have been coaching people for twenty-five years and most recently executives, entrepreneurs, and high performers on their health. There are many common traits that my clients exhibit, but the one that stands out is that they all want to get the edge to be their best. They are willing to sacrifice many things -- be it money, waking up early, or partying to get to the next level. When people come to me, it is to improve some aspect of their health. It could be stress reduction, improve health or look better. The reason doesn't matter all that much. The bottom line is when they get to me they are ready and will do what it takes to get better.

I get labeled a few different things, health coach, trainer, life coach (hate that one), fitness coach, or just coach. The funny thing is they are the same, but the theme always comes back to "Coach." My website says, "Executive Health Coach," and when I look at it even I sometimes wonder is that what I am or if that is what I do? It doesn't matter. At the end of the day I help people be the best version of themselves. How do I do it? I don't do anything. I help my clients see they have everything they need to be precisely what that is; they only need to act on it. In my case, it's usually related to health.

Let me take a step back and give the sixty-second version of how I got to be here. I have been an athlete my entire life and attended college to play baseball. My career was cut short due to injuries and simply put, I needed something to do to fill the void of not being able to play college baseball. This led me to the fitness industry and personal training.

I learned everything regarding being the best personal trainer I could be. I relentlessly studied exercise and nutrition. I was the best at it in my area and was way ahead of the completion which ultimately led me to work for a national company traveling around training trainers. I was on the corporate side of the industry. I was lucky to learn a ton of information about the business. I eventually left that and had a highly successful personal training studio that I opened with my wife. She is a certified holistic health coach and much smarter than me☺. About this time I shifted my education toward human psychology and performance.

This was when things changed for me. When I shifted my focus to psychology and performance, I started to see the connection between health and happiness, health and stress, and health and work satisfaction. I also noticed that I could give two people with the same starting statistics and goals the same plan and see one get results while the other received zero results. Why? It was their mindset and habits --As a result, I spend the majority of my time with clients working on those critical areas.

Do I still talk about workouts and nutrition? Of course, but only to make sure it's part of the plan. I have written thousands and thousands of workout plans and nutrition plans. I don't do that anymore. Why? To be honest, there are way smarter program designers out there than me. I hire a coach to write mine. My specialty is helping you DO the program and help you to FOLLOW the nutrition plan. And, that my friend starts in the melon right between your ears called a brain.

Why am I still passionate about health and fitness after all these years (been at this for over 25 years)?

As cliché as it may be, if you don't have your health, you have NOTHING! The older you get, the more this rings true. When I see the health status of people in and the way they treat their bodies like a dumpster fire, quite frankly, it pisses me off; and I want to change that.

Even if I can only be a small part of that change for others, I am good with that. My hope is that you read this book and find one to two things which have a positive impact on you to live your best life and put your health first. That's it, nothing too sexy; if you get more than that than hallelujah! However, I will still take one to two things.

I truly wish you, health and happiness.

Damon Moschetto
St. Augustine, FL
August 6th, 2019

1. A Simple Way to Look Awesome That Works for Busy Professionals

Who the heck doesn't want to look and feel awesome? Exactly, everyone does. Let's find out how simple it can be, shall we?

What is the difference between people who look and feel awesome, daily versus people who struggle to fit health into their life? I don't want to simplify the answer to much because while everyone is different, typically there are some common traits that we see people do to succeed.

The first thing is that it is a top VALUE for them. When you ask them about their values, health is listed in the top three with no room for negotiating, period. This makes it easier for them to get out of bed and get that workout in or say no to that desert. It's that important to them. For people who are out of shape and want to make a change, their value system must change too. Health has to move up the ladder.

The second thing is they have some type of accountability. When starting out trying to change habits having someone, whether it is a friend or coach to hold their feet to the fire, so i

to speak, makes a huge difference. Interestingly enough, it's not just beginners who get a coach. Top performers who want to keep that edge or make improvements are never afraid to get that help they need to excel. Obviously, if you are starting out getting help to get started is a no brainer, but I believe at some point everyone can use one for a time. Look at top athletes, they have a coach for all different areas of their lives, and that's why they are the best.

The last thing I will touch on today is discipline. This is a scary word for many people, but it shouldn't be. It doesn't mean you have to be like a drill sergeant but having the discipline to do things you don't want to when you should oftentimes is the difference between success and failure. The quote, "Pay now or pay later," comes to mind.

2. You Have to Pay Attention!

Where are you in your life and health? How did you get there? These are simple questions but often ignored for too long making it real hard to course correct.

For example, have you all of a sudden gained 20-30 pounds compared to where you were in high school or college? This is a simple example of not paying attention and is no different than running up a credit card.

Let's look at money and how you can compare it to losing or gaining weight. Everyone knows that if you spend more than you make you are going to eventually be in big trouble. It can lead to racked up credit card debt or even as bad as filing for bankruptcy.

Gaining weight is not that different from running up or maxing out your credit cards. How does it happen? Lots of reasons. You couldn't say no to that new television or that new outfit and you did it more than once.

You justify in your mind that you can pay it off, but low and behold, six months later, you are carrying a massive balance on your credit card and where it goes from there depends on if you decide to change.

This is no different from weight loss. You eat what you want when you want, hit happy hour regularly and boom you look up, and you have put on ten to fifteen pounds. There isn't much of a difference between the two examples.

It's a choice. Tony Robbins is famous for saying your destiny is based on your decisions or something like that, but I digress.

Here is the simplest way to fix the problem, but this word is where most people say, "Nope."

Here it is, you must have the DISCIPLINE to say no to that purchase and to say no that desert or happy hour.

We are in a time where saying no is not in style, and it can be very difficult.

I will leave you with this. You can pay now, or you can pay later, it's your choice.

3. Do Not Listen to It!

It's always there, that voice telling you, "It's ok to skip today's workout," and "It's okay to eat that junk; I earned it."

The voice is always there, it never goes away, but it does come less and less if you refuse to listen to it.

I will give you an example. I am traveling for some work, and I started a new workout program days before that is very specific, and it builds on each week.

After traveling and working, when I got to my hotel, it could have been effortless to skip my exercise until tomorrow or justify not doing it. Let me tell you there was a voice telling me to do exactly that.

So, what did I do? I changed and hit the hotel gym. The first thing I did was decide if I was going to pay for a day pass at a gym or if the hotel gym would work. I knew I could make the hotel gym work and went and got it done.

Did I have to modify a few things? Sure, but nothing bad enough to throw me off the program.

There are a couple of points here.

1. We all get that voice of why we don't need to follow through on whatever endeavor we are embarking on. It will always be there.

2. The way to combat it is taking immediate action as soon as the voice starts talking. If I had waited and decided to do some more work and do it later I guarantee I would have skipped it.

This is true in just about anything in life. We as humans want the path of least resistance. NOTHING great comes from taking the easy way out ever. You might feel good in the short term, but you are a loser in the long run.

4. WTF With Cardio? Still!

It still amazes me today with all of the research and top coaches, scientist, nutritionist, etc. available that the default workout for most people is still cardio.

I traveled recently and worked out in the hotel gym. I was the only one in there at first, but soon after, an overweight middle-aged dude came in and jumped right on the elliptical for twenty minutes and left. Five minutes later, an overweight younger woman came in and jumped on the treadmill to walk.

Now let me say first the fact that people are doing something active that is potentially good for them should be applauded. That being said, with seventy percent of the population being overweight choosing cardio as your first action is a mistake.

There are two things at play here when you look at the number of people who are overweight or obese:

1. People do not do anything at all. Eating healthy is not part of what they do, and any type of exercise is nonexistent.

2. They chose the wrong form of exercise or diet (for them) that gets no results and this in most cases is not their fault

Let's tackle number one. What is there to say here? You're overweight, unhealthy, and you know it, yet you choose to ignore it. I am a libertarian. That means I don't care what you do just leave me alone and I will leave you alone (simplified it a bit close enough). Here is the problem in this instance. When you don't take responsibility for your health you will become a drain on our society's resources. This may not be very politically correct, but it's a fact. If I end up having to pay with my tax dollars to keep you alive, I am going to be pissed, but if you're sick and unhealthy and it doesn't affect anyone else this is your choice; so, have at it.

Now for number two. This is either not paying attention or just doing what you are most comfortable doing. There have been mounds of research supporting strength training and maintaining or increasing muscle that helps losing weight and fat better than cardio. There is no one size fits all here and by no means am I saying there is, but the fact remains resistance training should be first on your list with cardio following. Nine times out of ten this is not the case. Are more people strength training than ever before? Sure they are, but still most people's default is cardio.

Here is the thing, I have been in the fitness industry my whole adult life and coached thousands of people, but there are millions of people that do not have coaches that join gyms and go right to the cardio deck.

Here is the difference fifteen to twenty years ago, this information wasn't available like it is today. You can google anything you want to know. If you google best exercise to lose fat, I guarantee strength training is on the first page.

From here it can get tricky, and you may need a little more help here but having said that stop using cardio as the default to losing fat. Should you do cardio? Yes, you should, just not as the priority.

This is a little simplistic, but maybe that's what we need right now. Please keep it simple but do what works for you.

If you have been doing cardio as the priority for years and your body is not where you would like it to be maybe you should change? Just a thought.

5. Traveling Can Be Brutal!

I know many people who travel for a living. I traveled for ten years every week and am now back on the road about five times in a quarter of the year.

When I traveled, every week several years back, I had to check myself not to go off the deep end and become unhealthy; ironically enough while working for a nutrition company. It's very easy to completely lose your health and fitness if you are a road warrior.

I think there are three keys to staying healthy on the road:

1. Plan your food.
2. Make sure you work out or at least move, and
    3. Get good sleep.

These may seem elementary, but when you do it all the time, it's not; trust me. By the way, I am writing this while I am on an airplane.

Food without a doubt is the biggest challenge because you are at the will of airport food or if driving what is available at various exits, etc.

Here are the snacks I eat while on the road. While I am not a fan of packaged food in general, when traveling, sometimes it has to happen so try and make the best choice and usually choose the following:

- Beef Jerky
- Water- tons
- Low carb bars
- Nuts

Having these available can keep you from getting too hungry and making a bad food choice or hold you until you can get to a good store or restaurant you can eat healthy food.

If I am near a health food store, such as Whole Foods or something similar, I buy food when I get there and have it on hand.

My go-to restaurants are Chipotle, Panera and Starbucks. I know Starbucks seems terrible considering all the crap they sell, but you can make a good choice here. For example, they sell decent bars. Get a tall Latte and a bar, and you have a three hundred-calorie breakfast or lunch that is not horrible. Could it be better? Sure, but sometimes you need to make the better bad food choice. With Chipotle and Panera, I know that the meat is at least hormone-free and decent. Again, not great; but it's a Hell of a lot better than going to olive garden and destroying a bowl of breadsticks.

With food, you have to be diligent in your choices as this will make or break you.

Next up is working out. Think about this for a second. You travel thirty to sixty minutes to the airport to arrive two hours before your flight. The only thing you do is sit in the airport waiting for your flight. Then you sit for two to three hours on a plane depending on your destination and layovers. Next, you drive to your hotel or destination.

If you do not at least go to the hotel gym and walk for twenty minutes or go to a gym and workout, you are a jackass plain and simple. Too harsh? Maybe, but seventy percent of the population is overweight, possibly more. You have to move your body and when I say twenty minutes on a treadmill that is the LEAST you should do. I prefer some metabolic conditioning that you can get done in twenty minutes but DO something. Just about all hotels have gyms these days, so no excuse not to.

Last is sleep. This one is underrated. Unfortunately, studies show that we do not sleep well in hotels because our brain doesn't shut off as it does in our own home or environment. This is WAY more technical, but trust me on this one and look it up if you don't believe me. There is a lot to this, but I will give you a couple of key things to consider. The first thing you want to do is to shut off all extra lighting in the room. This means cover up the clocks, shutoff nightlights, and make sure you draw the blocking shades. This seems trivial, but it is not. A straightforward fix for this is for you to bring an eye mask and wear it at night.

Next, make sure you shut off the television an hour before you go to sleep. If you are really into it, bring earplugs to block out the external noises that we all hear in hotels.

There is more you can do to hack your sleep, but this too will make a big difference.

Traveling can be a challenge to stay healthy, but not if you are intentional in your approach. If it's important to you it will happen.

6. The Inmates Are Running The Asylum

It seems like more than ever right now you have to pick a camp when it comes to health and fitness.

For nutrition, it's, are you keto? Vegan? Carnivore? Paleo?

For working out it's, do you do CrossFit? Yoga? Orange Theory?

Everyone seems to be choosing sides, and in nutrition it's the worst. Vegans and carnivores literally hate each other.

I am also leaving out the fact that the majority of the population eats absolute crap and doesn't exercise at all. I swear even these people are wearing that like a badge of honor. Yeah, that's right; I am unhealthy and love it. Okay, to each his own.

I have news for all the nutrition and workout zealots. There is no one size fits all approach. Period!

I believe in certain principles, but the fact is that if we cut out processed food, ate more vegetables, sustainable meats, and cut calories, overall, we would be healthier as a society without a doubt.

Do this first and then find what works for you.

Create healthy habits.

However, do not get sucked into the diet or workout dogma; it will not end well.

7. Environment Determines Your Outcome

The environment does determine your outcome. This is often overlooked or brushed aside as not that big a deal, but the environment you are in has a massive impact on how you perform or if you succeed in any endeavor.

How is your environment set up?

Are there healthy food choices in your kitchen?

Have you taken out all the crappy food in your house?

Do you have a gym in your house? Is the gym close to your home or work?

What have you done to make it easy for you to fit in your workout?

Most people can't answer these or don't care and wonder why they are out of shape.

The simplest thing you can do is set your environment up to be healthy.

Have healthy food and snacks available. Have a few kettlebells, a workout mat, a foam roller, and some bands in your garage or extra bedroom.

Most people have food that they know they shouldn't be eating all around their house, but wonder why they can't eat healthily? Willpower doesn't work. They have proven this.

The way you set up your environment makes the difference.

8. The Grind

Life is a grind

Life is hard.

Life is difficult.

In today's society, these are things that we don't like to hear.

As parents, we try to expose our children to as little difficulty as possible. We don't want them exposed to anything hard. We want to make it easier for them. I think that is human nature, not criticizing anyone here.

I don't think it's anyone's fault necessarily; it is just the current evolution of things.

To me, Rocky summed life up the best.

> "Let me tell you something you already know. The world ain't all sunshine and rainbows. It's a very mean and nasty place and I don't care how tough you are it will beat you to your knees and keep you

there permanently if you let it. You, me, or nobody is gonna hit as hard as life. But it ain't about how hard ya hit. It's about how hard you can get hit and keep moving forward. How much you can take and keep moving forward. That's how winning is done!"
— **Sylvester Stallone, Rocky Balboa**

This is the absolute truth. Life has always been hard since the beginning of time. The true warriors are the ones that rise to the challenge throughout history and are successful not just in their own life but in many instances in lifting others as well.

When you look at successful people of today, and from the past, they all have one thing in common -- they were able to overcome major obstacles and keep going even when things looked bleak.

Most people quit as soon as things get hard. That is the difference between winners and losers, and it is a metaphor for life.

Now apply this to your lifestyle. Are you healthy? Ideal weight? If you had to do something physical, could you do it?

You see most people want to be in great shape, but it is WAY too much work and sacrifice. Eating crap and not working out is more important.

Winners play the long game. Losers paly the short game. They need immediate gratification.

At the end of the day, if you don't have your health, you have nothing, but most people ignore this until it is too late.

Don't be like most people; don't be average. Be willing to sacrifice today to enjoy life for the long haul.

I am not saying to be super rigid and never have fun. So if that is what you think, that is complete copout.

It's as simple as picking your spots. When are you going to let loose and when are you going to reign it in? Where is the balance? You know where it should be.

Do you have goals? Are you tracking progress in certain areas of your life, or are you letting your life be ruled by your boss, and shitty circumstances?

Once you accept that life is a grind, and when you embrace it, things get easier; trust me.

9. Raise Your Standards

If you are not living a healthy lifestyle but would like to, why haven't you? Try and answer this honestly.

Most people wish they were in better shape. The wanted they lost weight. They wished they had more energy.

Thinking about it from this perspective is almost a guarantee for failure.

Wishing, wanting, and trying in this instance is the same thing. It never works.

How do you make that transition from wishing to doing?

I believe it is as simple as raising your standards. We all have them for all areas of our lives. If you are successful in any area of your life, it is because you have a high standard for that particular thing.

If you look at people who are successful in any area of their life be it health, relationships, money or career they have a certain standard that they adhere to that allows them to reach or maintain success in that area.

When you look at someone, who is in great shape, you might say, "They have no life," or "they don't have any fun."

Is this true? Maybe for a few, but for most, this is not true and unfair judgment.

They just have a standard that they adhere to.

What if you had that same standard?

Would you be at your ideal weight?

Would your health be better?

Would you have more energy?

The answer is most likely, "Yes."

This applies to all areas. Look at someone wealthy. Are they lucky? Unless they inherited their money, I would say, "No." They have a high standard for the financial station in life.

I do think there is one key ingredient to raising your standards -- belief.

Believe you can do it. Believe you are worth it. You have to have this.

When you combine a belief that you can do something with raising your standards, you can accomplish just about anything you focus yourself to do.

Don't believe me.

Look at successful people in any area of life and tell me they don't have high standards and believe in themselves. You can't.

10. Nutrition Nonsense

Nutrition is a trigger word in health circles today and is one of the most significant debated topics to being in shape or healthy.

This is the toughest part of this whole deal.

Ready?

No one diet works for everyone.

Sorry if you are vegan, paleo, keto, carnivore, etc. There isn't. Look at the research.

I have listened to debates between vegans and paleo/low carb scientists/doctors, and all they do is throw research back at each other saying their right.

The only thing they agree on is to eat non-processed crap, but that is about it.

One thing for sure is that it is the best place to start, stop eating crap.

I think you need to take three things into account when finding out what the best way to eat is for you.

To find out what works sometimes it's about elimination and addition to find out if it genuinely does work.

So here we go:

1. How do you feel? Truly feel. Lots of energy or none? Journal about this and keep track.
2. Stick to a plan for at least thirty days uninterrupted.
3. Eliminate all junk and limit alcohol.

Most people will say a particular way of eating doesn't work for them but never even come close to the three tips I just mentioned.

If you want to get lean and feel good, nutrition is going to determine this; so, isn't it worth taking at least thirty days to figure it out?

11. This is Awesome!

In a world filled with negativity, let's focus on something positive today, shall we?

Did you wake up in a house with electricity?

Do you have running water?

Do you have access to food?

Did you wake up in a house?

If you did, guess what? You are lucky compared to a LARGE percentage of the world.

Did you know that if you make $32,400 per year, you are in the top one percent worldwide (not US)?

So, what's the point? The point is it's not as bad as you think.

We live in a time where the media is always telling you that you are oppressed by someone, or something.

It's so easy to get bought into it.

I see people on social media with Masters Degrees, and Ph.D.'s constantly crying about hard it is for them and how things are unfair blah, blah.

Meanwhile, the person who has half the education they do are hustling providing massive value to other people and making tons of money.

The point? It's all about your attitude toward your individual circumstances.

If you are not happy with your job, get a new one. Currently, we are at almost four percent for the unemployment rate, and businesses are dying for good people to work for them

If you are overweight, change it.

The good news in all of this is you can practically be or do whatever you want.

We are living in a time when you can. Take advantage of it!

This is a time where things are pretty much at your fingertips if you want them.

Go get yours!

12. This Happens Every Year

We are at the end of 2019, and that means it's time for resolutions and new goals you set in place to transpire. Haven't you sat on yours for too long?

While I am a big fan of setting goals, resolutions have never made much sense to me. Waiting until the New Year to make positive changes seems counterintuitive to me.

So, what is going to be different this year?

The big joke is that the gyms will be full for a month and then empty again. It's sad but true, happens every year like clockwork.

Ask yourself, has this been you in the past? You start like gangbusters only to quit after a few weeks.

Alternatively, even if you do work out regularly, but you are not where you want to be physically or even mentally. How is this not going to happen this year?

How are you going to stick to this for the long term?

Here is one mistake I think people make during this time. The goals they set are too short term in thinking even if they think they are for the long run.

If you want to lose twenty pounds and keep it off, do you know the best time frame for this would be? A month? Twelve Weeks?

The correct answer is at least a year. Will it take you a whole year to lose twenty pounds? Maybe, maybe not, but the point is you want to keep it off. That means the entire year, not just twelve weeks or a month to lose weight.

The point is that goals need to be for the long term. It's not just about hitting the target but maintaining it.

When you take the long approach, it makes it much easier to stick to the plan because when you don't lose ten pounds in a week it does not phase you because you know there is plenty of time.

If you think you should be at your goal in a month and see little progress it becomes so easy to quit.

Most people don't have this, but there needs to be some patience applied to the process.

There is a little bit more to this, but I hope you get a general idea.

If you have any questions on this, please let me know!

13. What's The Secret?

It's the little things that count. No one likes to hear that.

Little things like:

- Getting adequate sleep.
- Drinking enough water daily.
- Having a plan to move daily.
- Planning out your food.

These seem trivial, but they are not.

Most people are online googling the greatest fat-blasting workout or the seven-day diets to lose one hundred pounds -- all ridiculous, but sexier to do than get eight hours of sleep every night.

That is the problem with most people that set fitness goals. They do not want to focus on the basics.

Why? Not flashy enough.

Most people want to be able to say, "Yeah, I am a Vegan now," or "I am doing CrossFit five days per week." That's sexy.

I get eight hours of sleep, watch my calories, and move daily, not sexy.

The sad part is the person that goes Vegan or does CrossFit like an asshole (you know the obnoxious ones that's all they talk about) lasts three weeks and quits while the non-sexy person sticks with the simple program for the year and loses twenty to thirty pounds.

What I am talking about here is the basics, and no one likes to hear it. You must master the basics in anything you are trying to be successful doing.

When you look at the people that are healthy and at their ideal weight, I guarantee they do the little things. The little things are different for everyone depending on where you are starting, but it still has to be done.

Master the basics day in and day out and before you know it people are asking you, "What's your secret"?

14. Routines

I talk a lot about routine and habits, but I do for a reason, they work.

If you want to live a healthy lifestyle, it starts with your morning routine. It's redundant, but the adage, "Win your morning, win your day," is true.

I recommend that my clients take inventory of how they start their day. Is it chaos or do they have a ritual?

I can personally attest to that when I skip my routine or get off my routine for a few days, I am almost always less productive.

Here are some common elements of a healthy lifestyle that will be omitted when the morning is chaos:

- Skip workouts. • Skip Breakfast.
- Do not plan the day's food.
- Don't drink enough water.
- Let email rule their day.

- Start their day lost in social media.

I could go on, but you get the point.

I firmly believe everyone needs to implement a morning routine which includes some movement, lots of water, meditation or prayer, gratitude journaling, and planning of day.

There is no right way, but you need to have one.

I have experimented over the years and found what works for me. I switch it up from time to time as well depending on what I have going on in my life at that time.

There is plenty of "Guru's" selling the magic way to do it. It's bullshit. There is no right way.

I have my opinion and help people create these regularly, but I help my clients find what works for them. Some people need two hours in the morning, and others are fine with twenty minutes.

Find what works for you, but you have to be intentional with your mornings.

I promise if you start a morning routine it will change your life for the better.

Let me know if you need some help with this.

15. Don't Repeat The Same Mistakes

If you were to look at your health and fitness from a year ago versus today, what would it look like to you?

Is it better or worse?

Worse is what I find with many people, even people that go to the gym regularly.

Why? Nothing changes.

Let me give you two examples.

Example one: Person A decides they are going to lose weight. They plan to join a gym and go on a diet.

Example two: Person B has been going to the gym for years and has been gradually gaining weight (this happens all the time). The plan is to go on a diet.

What is the outcome for these two? They both quit within six weeks.

Person A made no other changes to their life, so to try and fit something new it was an abysmal failure.

Person B bought a book and tried to wing it. Again, abysmal failure.

I could go into greater detail on each, but there is no need.

These two people did this exact same thing last year and the year before.

They decided to set a goal with no "why" behind it.

No real plan. Deep down inside, they knew they were not going to hit their goals.

Next year they will be setting the same goal.

How can you avoid this?

Write your goal down right now. Go ahead. I will wait.

Now next to it write why it's important for you to hit this goal. Do it with some passion behind it? Feel how good it feels when you achieve this goal.

Now write next to that how you will not settle for failure no matter how long it takes, you will hit this goal. You fired up? You should be. That's how you hit goals. Get excited about them! Want them more than anything.

Tony Robbins has a saying that goes something like this, "People are not lazy, they simply have impotent goals. That is goals that do not inspire them."

I think this is true if you are not inspired by your goals you won't hit them.

Get inspired!

16. Mindset Baby!

What are you focused on? This is the question you need to ask yourself daily.

Most of the time, the answer to this is trivial stuff that moves you no closer to your goals.

Are you checking social media every five minutes wasting twenty minutes a pop? I have, we all have, and we need to cut it out.

It takes discipline to stay on task, but if you want to move the needle forward in life you have make sure you are spending time on things that matter.

Did you do the things you need to do to stay healthy or reach your fitness goals today?

Did you learn something today? Did you get better at your craft?

If the answer is no, commit today to change that. It doesn't have to be anything over the top. In fact, it could be something as simple as going for a walk or reading something in your field for twenty minutes. If your answer is, "I don't have time," I call bullshit.

I think out of all the excuses we have, not having enough time is the biggest lie of all. Whenever my clients say this, and we take inventory of their day, we always find a minimum of two hours where they can be working towards something better.

Please keep this in mind, if you want something to change in your life, you must be willing to make the changes in your day to day to see improvement.

You can't keep doing the same thing day in and day out, which is usually nothing, and expect to make progress.

You can do this! You can get better! Change something today you know you have been putting off.

17. Hang With Lions Not Sheep

Level Up!

I think this is one of the most underrated concepts when trying to get better in life or reach any goals you set.

Many people I work with have goals they set for themselves, but when we evaluate whom they spend the majority of their time with those people are the antithesis of what they are trying to achieve.

Let me give you a quick real-world example.

Client A wants to clean up their diet, and a big part of that is cutting out or down their alcohol intake. The first thing we did was look at when and who she was with when this was happening. Unfortunately, the time she spent with her peer group almost always was spent around drinking.

This was eye-opening but created quite a challenge. Think about it. Imagine knowing you need to change to get better but all the people you spend your free time with do that thing you need to give up. This is where people usually give up but not my clients ☺.

So how did she do this without cutting everybody out? A few ways.

The first thing she did was start meeting her friends for coffee and skipping the happy hours. She even asked some to go for walks with her. This solved two things

1. It allowed her to still spend time with her friends but avoid alcohol or the temptation of it.
2. She was able to get a little bit of extra activity in.

I am not going to lie and say it was super easy or she didn't get any pushback because she did, but on the whole, it wasn't nearly as bad as she thought it was going to be. The side benefit she received from this was she found out who her true friends were. The ones who were always giving her a hard time she cut out of her life. The crazy thing was when I asked her if she missed those people, she said, "Crazy enough no I don't."

And, by the way, she didn't quit drinking alcohol; she had it when she wanted to, but was in control, and it wasn't the only thing she did with her peers. Sometimes she went out and drank and sometimes she didn't.

One thing she did do was upgrade her friend's. She found some new friends who were into fitness and being healthy. They did active stuff on the weekends. She even went to weekend retreats on Yoga and fitness. Something she could NEVER seeing herself doing.

Why?

She leveled up. She knew she wanted more and found out that getting around a better environment made a big difference. The beauty of this was that she kept her old friends and upgraded at the same time.

This is not nearly as hard as you think it is but you must have a clear intent about what it is you want.

It may be hard at first, but before you know it, you hit that goal you want, and life is even better than you could have imagined.

What are you willing to change to get better? What are you ready to give up?

18. Do It Even When You Don't Feel Like It!

When you do something, even when you don't feel like it, it separates the winners from the losers.

The winners do it even when they are tired.

The winners get it done when they have no time.

The winners get it done when it seems impossible.

Losers roll with the excuses and feel like crap because of it.

When you turn your should into musts, you will get rid of the excuses.

This takes one hundred percent commitment, which means that you will get that workout in you have scheduled even when your day gets messed up. It also means you will not eat crap just because you are too tired and busy.

It may sound like positive mumbo jumbo, but it's not. It's a fact. The most successful people will not allow excuses in their lives.

I have a rule. I work out in the morning. Before I go, I may be doing something, but as soon as a voice in my head says, "You are too tired," or "You can skip and go tomorrow," I immediately stop what I am doing and go to the gym.

Why? Because I know if I take too long I will give in to that voice in my head and skip it.

Whenever you hear that voice in your head say something contrary to your goals or what you know you should be doing, stop, and do that thing immediately.

19. Extreme Ownership

Have you ever wondered what separates the successful versus non-successful people?

Is it because they have better parents?

Went to a better school?

Came from money?

Maybe.

However, how many rich losers do you know? I know plenty, and their parents are still taking care of them.

When you peel away all the circumstances, the one thing that separates success from failure is ownership.

There is a book on leadership called *Extreme Ownership,* and I highly recommend you read it. It is written by two former Navy Seals who take their lessons learned in combat and apply them to life and leadership. At the book's core it's about taking one hundred percent responsibility for everything that happens in your life.

Imagine if you did that, how much better off would you be?

Would you be in shape? Yes.

Would you make more money? Yes.

Would you have better relationships? Yes.

Pick any area of your life, and it would be better.

By no means am I perfect when it comes to this, but the book had a significant impact on my life, and it is a principle I try and live every moment of my day.

Give it a shot and everything will change.

20. The Struggle is Real

Doing the right thing is hard. There is no way around it.

I think without a doubt, nutrition or eating clean is the hardest thing to do if your mind is not right.

We are bombarded daily with all these good looking foods, desserts, and alcohol, etc. and ninety-five percent of the people you are around are partaking. It's a challenge, to say the least.

Some people may disagree with me, but working out is the easy part, sticking to a nutrition plan is at least five times as hard in my humble opinion.

Think about how hard it can be if you are out with people at the latest coffee and dessert shop. All of your friends are getting cheesecake, cookies, chocolate cake, etc. and you say, "No." There is nothing fun about that.

Let's look at losing weight. For example, you are following a specific diet; when you do that, it's typically based around calories and macros.

To do this, you have to take the time to plan things out, so you make sure you stay on your plan. Makes sense right? Well in today's fast-paced society, that is a considerable challenge.

Most people will not commit to doing what they need to do to stick with it.

The people that do commit choose to because they have burned their boats and said I am doing this no matter what. What do they do? They do four things:

1. Decide
2. Commit
3. Create a strategy/plan
4. Implement the strategy/plan relentlessly

The method is much easier than you think, but it has to be thought out and acted on for it to be effective. Most people fail because their strategy sucks, saying, "I am going to eat better," is not a strategy. Saying I am going to eat X number of calories per day, four meals per day and I am going to research the best food services to make it fit into my busy lifestyle is a much better strategy. We could go much more in-depth on this, but you get the point.

I am not going to sugarcoat it for those people who are trying to implement a healthy lifestyle. It takes commitment and trial and error to make it stick, but you HAVE to see it through.

Is it easier for me? Sure, but I have been working at this my entire adult life. I have put in the time, so it's effortless for me to say no to dessert and booze. By the way, I do eat dessert and drink occasionally but, on my terms, not anybody else's and that's the difference. I don't give a flying crap what anybody thinks about me at a social event saying no, and most people can't do that.

Seriously, think about this for a minute. I have had clients say to me that they could never say no to eating or drinking at a social event as it may upset people. What? Are you serious? Who gives a shit? It's your life, and maybe that's why you're fat?

Did I offend you with that last line? If I did you should think about it again because everything I just said is on point and you can either make changes or stay fat, your choice.

Sometimes we need a hard dose of the truth to make changes. God knows I do; ask my wife ☺.

21. Tough Times

We all encounter days where we want to throw in the towel. You know, the ones that continuously throw garbage at you even when you are busting your ass.

It happens.

How we respond to those days is what matters.

If we let it drag us down before you know it, we have lost a month, and we feel bad about life.

Working out is the easiest example. If I miss a day of my workout, it is very easy to go to the gym the next day.

However, if I miss a week, forget it, the struggle becomes real! The further away you get from what it is you are supposed to do the harder it becomes to do it.

Here is something I do now when I feel like I don't want to do what I should. It goes like this:

I try and get outside if the weather cooperates and sit in the sun for five minutes and get in a state where I am open and calm and not irritated about what has been going on. Then I write down three things I am grateful for and mean it. Then I think of all the hugely successful people whom I admire and imagine what they would say to me. Most of the time, it works.

The bottom line is that you have to get out of the state you are in to move forward. If not, you get sucked into a vortex of negativity.

Another thing you can do is go to *YouTube* and search in "Motivation." There are a plethora of motivational videos you can watch that will get you moving.

No one is perfect. We run into struggles all the time and always will, but we must find ways to stick to things we know are good for us.

If you are in a place that I just described, make a commitment, to change today. I promise you will feel better even if it's your commitment is to take a ten minute walk to clear your head.

22. 80/20

We only have one life; this is a fact, but most people ignore this until something catastrophic happens in their life.

Today it has become more in vogue to party hard and deal with the hangover tomorrow. In other words, there is no longer a need to care about the body because "You only live once."

Then there is the opposite of that in which the only thing people focus on is working out, eating only organic food, taking supplements, and biohacking their health.

I think both of these approaches are wrong.

On the one hand, I lean more toward taking care of your body but at the same time that does not mean you can't ever party or have a piece of pizza.

I talk a lot about extremes, and this is just another example -- the all or nothing principle.

I have always lived by the 80/20 rule or 90/10, and it has served my clients and me well.

If you are healthy, and at your ideal weight or fitness level, that means that you need to live a healthy lifestyle, eighty percent of the time and can relax twenty of the time.

So, what does that mean? That means that going out to dinner on a Saturday night and having a few drinks is fine. You get back on the normal plan, and things are good. During the week you miss a workout due to family issues - - no big deal. You essentially stay on track, enjoy life but don't go off the rails and get unhealthy.

If you are unhealthy or have a weight loss goal, for example, you have to be tighter. There is not much room for error. In this instance you go out to dinner, and you make a healthy food choice. You then have to decide between dessert and alcohol - not enough room for both. The good news here is that once you hit that goal you get to switch to the eighty percent and you have more room to splurge.

When it comes to your health, you have to decide whom you want to be. You either want to move well, look good and feel good, or you don't.

If you don't, you may have a blast early on, but you will pay for it sooner than later. You see this all the time. You find out someone's age, and you thought, "I thought he or she was ten years older than they are" or "I thought they were ten years younger than they are." Along with the looks comes the health as well.

The person who looks older than they are, and the ones who don't are still competing daily.

It's a choice.

You can choose to find a balance between that party life and living a healthy lifestyle.

Whom you spend most of your time with will play a significant role in this choice.

Choose wisely.

23. Genetics?

Let me ask you a question.

Have you ever wondered why some people seem to be able to be in great shape no matter what or it looks like they eat whatever they want and still look great?

I think everyone wants to know the answer to this because we have all witnessed it

Before I answer this, think about where you are currently at with your health and fitness

Are you where you would like to be? What does your day look like?

The reason I ask this is that people are usually jealous of the person in shape while not even looking at their current situation.

We sometimes assume the person that is always in shape is just lucky or had great genetics.

Is that true? Maybe in some cases but I would argue that for most it's not the case.

So, let's look at the people that are always in shape and why that is.

I don't believe there is one specific reason that they can look good all the time.

First, a quick word about genetics. It has been said that sixty percent of our bodies are simply due to genetics which leaves forty percent to make improvements or go downhill.

Here is the deal, you can do a lot with forty percent either way. My argument regarding the forty percent is that people treat themselves like a dumpster fire and blame it on genetics.

Some examples of the sixty percent you cannot control are height, eye color, hair color, etc. However, you do have control over your emotions and how you treat your mind and body.

You can control how you feel emotionally spiritually and physically. You are in control of those things, not genetics.

So back to the original question, I have several answers, but the simplest one is to stop paying attention to those people because you have no idea what they actually do or if they are actually healthy!

Focus on you and becoming the best version of you. Control your forty percent and watch things fall into place exactly where you want them.

24. Are You Diligent?

Being diligent with anything valuable in your life is vital to your success.

Are you diligent when it comes to your health?

I bet you are when it comes to your kids or your job. So you may be thinking, well of course I am, those are extremely important.

You will not get much argument from me about their importance, but I will give you another way to look at it.

Anything in your life that is important such as your family or job are one hundred percent meaningless if you do not have your health.

Read that last line again.

So, I will ask you again, are you diligent with your health?

Do you work out daily?

Eat only nutritious foods daily?

Are you actively working on stress reduction?

Are you getting quality sleep nightly?

Are you eliminating the negative crap in your social media feed?

Are you turning off the twenty-four negative news cycle?

The bottom line is that most people are ignoring the fact that our physical and mental health are more important than everything else because without it you have NOTHING!

The good news is that if you start making health your number one priority everything else that is important in life gets better. If you haven't made this change, stop waiting, and do it today.

Time is our worst enemy. You cannot get it back. Stop wasting it on trivial shit that doesn't keep you healthy.

25. Dogma

Whenever someone tells me this is the only way that you can eat, workout, or be healthy, I am gone.

In other words, I don't do "Dogma."

When you look at anything in life that has something in it that preaches "the only way" it is usually followed by some bad shit.

Vegans can be very dogmatic, not all of them but certainly most that I have encountered. The early days of CrossFit were like this, but it has calmed down a bit.

By the way, I have nothing against either one of those. If they work for you, please, by all means, continue; however, if you look and feel like crap you have to be honest and maybe try something else.

I have tried many diets and workouts in my career, some with great success and some failures. Imagine if I bought into the ones that made me feel like crap, where would I be? Would I eventually get healthy, perform at my best or continue to decline?

The answer is obvious, and sometimes, it is somewhere in the middle.

Sticking with the Vegan theme (it's easy to contrast), it doesn't mean if that's not working that I go one hundred percent carnivore but, unfortunately, that is what many people do.

If you are a reader/follower of my stuff, you know I am a massive fan of the basics.

Rather than jumping to some complicated way of eating or workout, start with the basics, and master them.

At that point, if you feel the need to go in another direction or challenge yourself then take that next step, but not until then.

A better example of this, if you have been eating like crap for ten years, don't think you are going to flip a switch, go vegan, keto, paleo, or carnivore and believe you will be able to stick with it for more than a hot minute.

Get good at the little things over and over, get success, and then move on but avoid getting sucked into the Dogma.

I promise you that never ends well.

26. This Will Never Change

What is the most natural thing you can do to look and feel great?

I would argue that nothing is. Think about it for a minute, is anything great in life easy?

If you want to have a great relationship, you work at it.

If you want to be good at your job, you work hard.

If you want a raise, you work hard and go the extra mile, so your boss recognizes your effort.

Being a good parent takes patience, and work has anyone on earth ever said, "I want to be a shitty parent," even bad parents would never admit or say it.

So why in the Hell would it be any different for looking and feeling good?

The point here is that anything in life worth doing has always taken hard work and always will.

The sooner you accept this and embrace it, the easier it is to get it done.

There is good news when it comes to looking and feeling great. It is simple and not complicated.

People don't get results because not only does it take work, but they complicate it with crazy diets and workouts. There is no need for that.

Keep it simple, be consistent, and you will be in great shape.

For some people, this is not what they want to hear. They want that magic workout or diet they are willing to do for thirty days to get a big payoff. I have a news flash for you; it doesn't exist!

My message is consistent and doesn't resonate with some because I speak the truth, and it's not sexy, but the ones that do, get results.

And, guess what? The people that do get my message become sexy ☺.

27. Motivation is For Pussies

We often look outside for motivation, and in some instances, I think it is excellent. For example, I think starting your day off with some motivational speeches or compilations is a great idea.

Having said that, if you only rely on external motivation, your will to succeed will never last.

External motivation essentially means whatever you are doing is for reasons other than your own. That is no Bueno.

The key to sticking to things long term and staying motivated long term is INTERNAL motivation. It has to come from you!

Why do you want to lose weight?

Why do you want to have more energy?

Why do you want to feel good?

Why do you want to look sexy? (There is nothing wrong with this)

These questions can only be answered by you. Answer these with strong why's and conviction. In other words, be excited about it and see yourself achieving whatever it is you want, but here is the trick.

See yourself doing the hard work, visualize getting through it no matter what and feel just how good those feelings are.

That is from you. That is what will keep you going when, "You don't feel like it," or "Are too busy."

We all need a little external motivation now and again but make sure that internal reason is close behind to keep it going for the long term.

28. Your Schedule is King

When it comes to our health, whether it is being healthy or merely wanting to look sexy, your schedule is a HUGE factor in you accomplishing that.

Do you schedule your workouts?

Do you schedule when you are going to eat? I know it sounds a little OCD, but stick with me on this one. If you look at most people, they either eat at the same time every day or are all over the place. If you know when and what you are going to eat how much better off will you be? You will be in charge of what's going in your mouth and when. That is a bigger deal than you may think.

Most people let their day be dictated by other people, or in many cases their email at work.

When you schedule your workout, you get it done.

When you schedule your nutrition, you make good choices.

When you schedule a time for important relationships, they improve.

When you schedule a time to read or for continuing education you improve on many levels.

Much of your success in life starts with your schedule.

Take control of it today and watch how everything improves and becomes more consistent.

29. You Have to Truly Want to be Healthy

When working with clients, I know within ten minutes if he or she will be successful in reaching their health and fitness goals. Why? A couple of reasons.

The first reason is the language that they use. If they talk a lot about past failures or use the word "try" more than once I know their odds of success are slim unless they make some serious internal changes. If they use words like "committed," or "I want to change," I know their chances of success are high.

The second reason is whom they spend most of their time. If their social circle is anti-health, it will be a challenge versus people that will support them.

This doesn't mean people can't be successful despite these circumstances, but it can make it harder or easier depending on where they are currently starting.

This may sound corny, but I think you need to wake up and know that being in shape, eating healthy foods is simply what you do. You make it part of your identity.

It doesn't mean it's "all" you are, but it is important that you make this part of your life day in and day out.

Imagine for a second, if you woke up every day with the intention of only doing things that make you feel outstanding both physically and mentally. What would that look or feel like?

How do you think that would play out in the long run?

How would you feel?

Would you get up ready to take on your day?

Most people do the exact opposite. They go right to social media, email, television, or any other useless negative crap.

We are bombarded with negativity all day long. The media wants us divided or wishing we had more of something we don't even need.

This may not be the most profound statement you will ever hear, but you have to truly want to be healthy, or it won't happen.

I don't believe there is a middle ground with this. You can bullshit yourself and say you are healthy when you're not, but we both know that is a lie.

It may not be easy at first, but if you stick with it the rewards on the other side are well worth it, trust me!

30. Did You Give Up?

At this point, no one would blame you if you did give up on being healthy.

Seventy percent of the population is overweight, and several diseases are caused by it, but the answer seems to be in a pill. The funny thing is that medicine causes you to need another pill.

There is a big debate over the cost of health care, which makes me laugh because we do not have a system that promotes health in the first place.

We are living in a time where it is so easy; we have lost sight of what it takes to work hard. What we think is hard today our grandparents laugh at.

So, it only makes sense that our health is going down the drain.

It's all about eating and drinking. That is all there is.

Look at marketing; it's either about food or booze.

If you don't drink today, you're the odd one out, and it makes people uncomfortable.

If you eat only healthy foods, you get an eye roll from other people.

Are you trying to be your best and hold yourself to a higher standard? That's crazy and a waste of time.

You should just fit it. Be like everyone else.

In other words, fit in with the rest of the sheep.

Or, you can do the opposite.

Work on you.

Commit to improving daily.

Ignore the losers who give you a hard time or lose them altogether.

Some people are okay being sheep and some people want to be the lion.

Be the lion.

Embrace the work.

It's fucking hard.

However, you earn your results, and it feels amazing, much better than it being handed to you.

That's the reward.

31. Simple, But Beautiful

I think it's the simple things that are sometimes the most poetic or pretty.

We live in a time where everything is all about the flash -- the sexy new phone, car, TV, computer, etc.

This applies to health and wellness more than ever.

A simple workout that gets results. Hogwash.

A simple eating strategy that you can implement regularly and get results. Not exciting enough for me because it will not look good on Instagram.

Don't get sucked into this; it's a lie.

Simple is sexy.

Simple gets results.

Simple is sustainable for the long term.

Simple can be done anywhere.

Simple isn't complicated.

Working out should be simple, not complicated.

Eating healthy should be easy; not a challenge.

If you are saying to yourself, "Being healthy is too hard to stick with," you are doing it wrong.

32. How Deep?

This scares people when you start to talk about more than just surface things.

When people (myself included) are having a difficult time in their lives, many times it is because they are not willing to do the deep internal work necessary to fix it.

When I say, "deep," it means something different to everyone depending on circumstances and situations. For example, when someone has gained weight consistently over a period of time, say two years, the easy thing to look at is nutrition and exercise.

In all my years of coaching, people rarely say that is the TRUE cause. The true cause or reason has more to do with what's going on inside, spiritually and mentally.

Here's the rub, as soon as you mention this to people they run for the hills. They want no part of facing the real challenge in their life. It's way too much work and too painful to face.

Of course, it's a lie. It's much worse in the long run when you do not confront the real issues in your life, and the longer you put it off; it makes it a much bigger challenge to overcome them.

Here are some example root causes:

Thirty-something-year-old mother who has a desk job and a couple kids has gained about thirty-five pounds over the past five years. On the surface it looks like she is super busy, drinking too much wine, eating junk and not exercising.

While all of those may be true, the real question you have to ask yourself is why? You and I both know she does not feel good about herself carrying an extra thirty-five pounds around and feels like crap.

In this instance, after digging in and having deep conversations, she is utterly miserable in her marriage and hates her job. How is she dealing with it? Eating and drinking and altogether avoiding the real issue.

Why? It's hard to face your crap that ultimately you and nobody else is responsible.

It's hard to have those tough conversations with a spouse or loved one.

It's scary to think about starting a new job.

I worked with many men who were financially well off, but miserable. These guys couldn't stand their wives so they golfed every day so they could waste five hours and not have to spend time with their wives. Most of them wouldn't divorce because of either how it looked or how much it was going to cost them financially.

I have worked with people that have the tough conversations and ones that don't. The ones that do, it's like ripping off a band-aid. It stings at first, but before you know it you are glad you did it.

The ones that don't sadly get worse. I am not unsympathetic when I say this, but they get fatter, sicker and unhappy. Moreover, by the way, many of these people exercise and use it as punishment.

We all have a choice. Most times, the tough decisions are the right ones to make that will make our lives better down the line.

You have to be willing to look inside of ourselves and get honest. Ask the tough questions and accept the tough answers.

And, then what? Take the right action!

33. What is Real Health?

What is health? Health means something different to everyone.

Let's define health from Webster's dictionary:

1. The condition of being sound in body, mind, or spirit
2. A condition in which someone or something is thriving or doing well: Wellbeing.

Based on the definitions above, health is so much more than how we look.

It's much more than working out and nutrition.

If you look at the first definition, the focus is on body, mind, or spirit. Most people only focus on the body.

Is that the true driver of health? I would argue that if mind and spirit are in a good place, health of the body will follow naturally, and if not, the body will suffer regardless of working out and diet.

I know, a little woo woo, but stick with me.

When I say naturally, "I don't mean doing nothing, and you will be in great shape," quite the contrary. If the mind and spirit are in line, the two will to take care of the body through proper nutrition and exercise will flow naturally. Sticking to your exercise plan becomes easy. Eating nutrient-dense foods becomes the norm.

A positive mind and spirit are different for everyone, and that is for you to find out. For me when I am managing stress well and consistent with my spiritual practice, I am on top of my mind and spirit. For some that means going to spending time alone to manage stress and going to church and praying. It doesn't matter what it is; there is no one right way.

I am not going to lie, managing my stress and spirit is way harder for me than working out and eating right. To be honest, I struggle with it a lot, but I also know that if I don't face it, it only gets worse and everything in my life suffers.

So, ask yourself, are you managing your mind and spirit? If not, what can you do today to make a change?

Start with something small. For stress, that could be taking a ten-minute walk focusing on breathing to relax. For spiritual, it could be reading a spiritual book that resonates with you.

Keep it simple, but if you are struggling with your body take a serious look at your mind and spiritual health first.

Love to hear your feedback on this.

34. Get Your Head in the Game

One of the most challenging things when it comes to your health is the fact that it is a daily, weekly, monthly, yearly battle.

It's not a twelve week endeavor.

As hard as this concept is to grasp, once you do and then embrace it, it's much easier to tackle head-on.

One of the things that makes this difficult is the health and fitness industry.

No one markets this concept.

They market seven-day cleanses and twelve-week transformations. I get it; I was guilty of this when I owned my studio.

Think about it, if a gym or personal trainers marketed lifetime commitment, how would that go over?

It wouldn't.

I think this is responsible for the rise of the $10 per month gyms. They know it's a hard sell, so they make it as cheap as possible. Most people that belong to these low-cost gyms spend more on coffee in two days than they do on the gym all month.

We all are only here for a short time. We can function optimally for as long as possible or fade away quickly.

Ten years go by in a blink.

In ten years, where will you be if you continue on the current path?

Hey look, we're all going to die, morbid I know.

How do you want to go out?

I see people living in their 80s who are being kept alive by meds and utterly dependent on other people.

I also see people in their 80s at the gym, golfing and independent.

It's all determined by what you do today and the next day.

The good news is that you are one hundred percent in control.

35. What Motivates You?

I write a lot about health and performance.

One of the biggest obstacles to health and performance often is lack of motivation.

It's safe to say we all have our moments of "not feeling it today" when it comes to our workouts or making healthy choices.

This is where it can be a slippery slope if you decide not to do what it was you were planning on doing be it training, writing, meditating, or reading.

Assuming you are doing these things to improve yourself either physically, mentally, or spiritually, most of your day is set up to do the exact opposite. That part is not your fault.

When we set up a routine or set a goal that is in pursuit of something greater than where we are currently or when you are on this path it is a challenge but gratifying.

The Stoics discuss this at length. Below are a few examples:

"No man is more unhappy than he who never faces adversity. For he is not permitted to prove himself." Seneca

"A gem cannot be polished without friction, nor a man perfected without trials." Seneca

"Man conquers the world by conquering himself." Zeno

We live in a time where we have never had it easier, and yet most people still think it's too hard. I am by no means immune to this, and I believe in our current age we all succumb to it.

I believe this is one of the main drivers of our obesity crisis. If it's hard, we don't do it. However, I digress.

Motivation has to come from within to be maintained in the long term.

The question is, what motivates you? Most people can't answer this.

Most people don't even know what they want, and therefore there is no motivation. Think about that for a second as it makes perfect sense. If you don't see what you want, how in the heck would you be motivated to stick with anything?

Before you start that exercise program, diet, or whatever endeavor you are embarking on get abundantly clear on exactly why you are doing it. If you do that the internal motivation will always be there or at least most of the time.

If you need help with; let's talk. Happy to help.

36. If the Word Health Meant Sexy

Health and wellness are boring. I wish it weren't, but it is.

Imagine for one moment if the coolest thing was being healthy.

That would mean that working out was the cool thing everyone did; healthy foods were the rage and getting to bed early was cool.

On the surface, you may be saying how boring. Maybe or maybe not.

Look at the other side. Most people work forty to sixty hours per week waiting for Friday so they can go out to eat and get drunk and repeat it on Saturday night. If you analyzed the typical person's week that is what it looks like. How do I know this? I coach these people. They come to me because they have finally woken up to the fact it's slowly killing them and there must be a better way.

I understand why they do it. Most work all week in either a job they don't like or a super high-stress job. It only makes sense that at the end of the workweek they want to escape, and alcohol and decadent food is easy to get.

Now you may be thinking does this mean I need to completely change. The short answer is Hell yes!

The long answer is to figure out precisely what you want, make a plan to get there, knowing that it will not happen overnight.

I used to sugar coat things and said you could be healthy and not impact your lifestyle that much. It was a lie that I even bought into trying to make it easier for my clients.

I don't think you can have it both ways. You have to choose a side. You are either going to be healthy or not.

I had a co-worker who owned being unhealthy, and to be honest; I respected it. She said I am fat and do not care about how I look or my health. She drank like crazy and ate tons of junk, but she owned it. The fact that she is unhealthy and on a bunch of meds is an entirely different discussion for a different day.

I can respect that more than the people who "want" to get in shape or are going to "try" and get to the gym.

Do it or don't. No one cares one way or the other.

I am fortunate enough to only work with people who are one hundred percent committed and do not deal with the people that are sitting on the fence being healthy one day and eating at McDonald's the next. This may seem harsh, but I promise it's not.

Why? Those people that commit get results, feel great, look great, and figure out how to work in the partying and social events without losing themselves but still have a blast.

At the end of the day, the one thing that rings true is anybody can get healthy and still have fun at the party. It's just finding a balance.

If you need help, let me know.

37. Are You a Million-Dollar Racehorse?

Are you a million-dollar racehorse? The obvious answer is no!

I read an article the other day talking about this, and it caught my attention. The credit goes to Joe Polish, but I speak about the same thing in different ways.

Think of yourself as a million-dollar racehorse.

If you owned a million-dollar racehorse, how would you treat it?

You wouldn't shove fast food down its throat.

You wouldn't cause it to have sleep deprivation.

You would make sure it gets the best trainers, the best tracks, and the best everything.

You would take care of that million-dollar racehorse because it needs to win races to make you money.

So, *YOU* are that million-dollar racehorse. If you treat yourself any other way, you are likely messing yourself up.

Part of this is about how you physically take care of yourself. It also involves whom you hang out with during your free time. Cut all ties with dishonest, lazy people.

Look at the environment in which you live and work. Is it supportive to be the best version of you?

Take a look at your business (work) and life and ask:

- Is your environment supportive?

- Are the people you associate with supportive of the way you want to live?

- Are you treating yourself in a way that makes your life healthy, productive and fun?

Treat yourself like the million-dollar Racehorse you are.

38. The Carrot or the Stick?

We all lack motivation from time to time, and it is NEVER a good feeling.

Here are some examples:

- Do not want to do that report for work.
- Don't feel like reading that book that will help further my career.
- Don't feel like cooking. O Don't feel like training.
- Don't feel like getting out of bed.
- And, the list goes on and on!

So, what do you do to get these important things done?

The subject line of this chapter said, is it the carrot or the

stick? I have good and bad news!

The good news is they both work! The bad news is that they both only work for a short time.

If you noticed the words I used above describing when we don't do things I started with "Don't feel like it," it should be a wakeup call for you.

So, there is the problem, the word "Feels."

This is going to sound harsh but Fu*k your feelings!

It is way too easy to listen to the voice telling you it's okay to not do X, Y, or Z.

That my friend is a slippery slope, you do not want to go down.

My best advice is that the second you hear that voice saying you, "Aren't feeling it today to do whatever you are supposed to," go and do it immediately.

Ask yourself how many times you justified something stupid you know you should have done and felt like crap for the rest of the day?

You don't need a carrot or a stick you need "done."

Seriously, do whatever it is right now. Don't wait or put it off.

39. Are You a Bad Motherfucker?

That's right. It's a serious question.

I don't care if you're twenty or seventy.

I love it when I see an older lady or gentlemen getting after it at the gym.

Why? Because they said to themselves, I don't care about age or anything else I am going to kick life in the dick.

Lately, I feel like we are being told to be, how do I say this?

A woos? A pansy?

I think it is one of the reasons we are reaching an all-time high in obesity.

We can't be a badass. Badass means something different to everyone, and it's all good! To me, it means you are going to get after it and not allow excuses in your life.

Work sucks! You still kick in the door and get it done.

Tired? You still go to the gym and crush it.

You want to have a great day? Default -- aggressive. Aggressive doesn't mean hurt people or anything stupid like that. It means you are going to move forward hard; but not reckless. There is a slight dichotomy with being aggressive but for today be aggressive.

You are still nice to people, but you don't tolerate excuses with yourself or anyone else.

Get after it.

40. Time Wasters - Are You Guilty of This?

There are many distractions vying for your time and attention. The number one thing to protect, as it relates to how well you work, is your attention and what takes up your attention is all the obligations.

People are too busy stepping over gold coins and picking up the bronze and silver coins. If you can identify the gold coins, and spend your time picking those up, it changes everything. So, what is a gold coin for you will not be a gold coin for someone else? Everyone has different gold coins.

This is so on point. It slapped me right in the face. I am guilty of this and needed it. Are you?

Time is the one thing we can never get back.

You can get money back.

You can get relationships back.

You can't turn back time.

Take inventory of where you are wasting your time.

The number one time waster today is social media followed closely by watching television.

Find your gold coins.

41. This is Simple, but Almost No One Does It

Are you having a hard time sticking to your nutrition plan?

Can you stick to your workout?

Can you stick to your professional development plan?

Get accountable. It is the easiest way to get and stay on track.

I honestly think it is the quickest way of accomplishing any goal you set.

Having someone that helps you stay on track and can call you on your bullshit excuses is a must if you want to be successful in any area in life.

Take a look at where you are falling short in life. Could you use some help? If so, hire a coach. If you can't afford a coach, ask a friend you trust that will give it to you straight to hold you accountable.

And, by the way, using the, "I can't afford it excuse to get results is unacceptable." There are different ways to get accountable.

If you truly want success in an area, you can make it happen.

42. What's Your Plan?

We all know that you have to work out and you know that I am a big believer in committing to some form of strength training.

The biggest challenge I see when working with people on their workouts is two things:

1. No plan.
2. Not tracking or measuring their progress.

When professionals go into a workout, they need a plan. Why? Simply, they have four hundred different things on their mind such as sales, presentations, making kids events, etc.

The last thing they need is their mind taxed trying to figure out what kind of workout they should do. That is why you see default to the treadmill or do a few strength machines and leave.

It's ineffective.

The other option is going to some class where unfortunately most of the time the goal is to get the crap beat out of you, and that's no good either.

So, to solve number one get on a program designed specifically for you and your goals.

If you get on the right program tracking your progress is key to making sure you are moving in the right direction or if you need to make some adjustments.

Thomas Monson said, "When performance is measured, performance improves. When performance is measured and reported, the rate of improvement accelerates. "

Are you increasing your sets? Weight? Changing tempo? If you are not tracking, you don't know if you are getting better.

If you think about it in any area of life, if you are not tracking how do you know if it's working or not? You don't.

These two things will make it way easier to get the results you desire.

43. The #1 Killer of High Performance

What is the number one killer of high performance these days?

In my humble opinion, it's stress.

Are there other factors such as nutrition, sleep, and recovery? Of course, but stress is the driver that kills performance.

How do you know if stress is ruining your performance? It's different for everybody, but a few signs are:

- Gaining belly fat.
- Trouble sleeping.
- Feeling fatigued all the time.
- Low sex drive.
- General loss of motivation.
- And, much more...

How do you fix it?

Again, different for everyone, but you want to do something called "working in" rather than "working out."

The last thing you want to do when stressed out is high-intensity workouts.

I would start with a thirty-day simple program centered on the following:

- No alcohol for thirty days.
- Start a SIMPLE guided meditation program (as little as five minutes a day).
- Go to bed thirty to sixty minutes earlier than usual.
- Eat only whole foods, cut out as much processed shit as possible.
- Drink a ton of water.
- Reduce caffeine intake to one cup a day.

There are ways to individualize this based on the person, but this would be a pretty simple and a solid way to reduce your stress and watch your performance go through the roof.

It's not rocket science, but most people complicate it enough that you would think it was.

If you are stressed, give this a shot.

44. Who Are You?

It's a legitimate question.

We all have identities we create. Some are good, some are bad. Are you a "healthy" person or something else?

I talk a lot about values and the fact that health needs to be a top-three to be your best.

This life is a gift.

Regardless of what you believe spiritually, I can't imagine we were put here to treat our selves mentally and physically like a dumpster fire.

I made up my mind years ago that health was something I would not sacrifice.

I want to be here for my family and not just be there but at a high level (at least high level for me ☺).

We all have a choice. I say this to my son all the time, "You can pay now or pay later, it's your choice."

It's solid advice. Why? Someone way more successful in life told me that a long time ago.

Think about how many times you put things off you know you should do and then later when there is no other option, and you have deal with it, it's way worse.

I see this with health all the time. People put on blinders and eat like crap, don't move, and before you know it, you're forty with health issues.

Don't be that person. Get your head right and make the tough choice of paying now so you can enjoy later.

It doesn't matter if you're thirty, forty, fifty, sixty, seventy, or eighty, make health a priority.

45. Action

Are you unmotivated?

Can't get to the gym? Eat right?

This is one of the most common excuses I get, "I know I should, but I just can't get motivated."

I will be honest, I have said that many times. In fact, I am a little ashamed about it.

Why? It's a complete bullshit excuse and an absolute lie.

Do you want the best antidote to lack of motivation? Take action. Get up and do something.

We live in this crazy world of needing to be motivated. Imagine two hundred years ago saying this.

People didn't live like that they took action, or they starved to death. We have it too easy.

No one wants to hear, "Take action." They want a magic plan.
There isn't one. You have to do the work.

Again, no one wants to hear that.

Do I coach people and work on plans with them? Of course, but if they don't do the work, the plan is useless. I usually fire those clients quickly.

46. Tons of Energy to Kickass in Life

If you think about that shouldn't having tons of energy be a top priority in your life? This is a no brainer. Tons of energy. Kickass in life.

If I gave you a plan that guaranteed this, would you do it?

Seventy percent of the people reading this wouldn't.

Seventy percent of the country is overweight. Could this number be high? Maybe. It's irrelevant because most people won't do the work.

Do you know that if you get eight hours of quality sleep, drank one hundred ounces of water, cut out alcohol, and moved your ass for an hour a day you would have tons of energy? Very few people will follow that SIMPLE advice.

I preach about the basics. Master the basics. That advice is basic.

Do you know why the basics are hard? They are somewhat boring and require commitment.

Listen, being healthy and looking good is not complicated; in fact, I would say it's simple but not easy. However, name me one thing in life that is great that doesn't require commitment and work?

You can't.

If you focus on the process consistently, the results will be amazing, I promise.

47. Tired, Sick and Miserable

I work with executives and entrepreneurs who are high performers in their careers but usually when they come to me; they are miserable and unhealthy.

They are incredibly frustrated because they are super successful in most areas of their lives but are a mess physically and sometimes mentally and emotionally.

The good news for these people is it's simple to get them on track. Why so simple?

I will water it down a bit, but basically, it has them look at the successes in their lives and uncover the habits and mindsets that allow them to flourish in those areas. We then apply that to their health.

It's different for everyone but it's not complicated.

Take a look at your health.

Are you healthy?

Ideal weight?

Feel comfortable at the beach or avoid it because you have to take your shirt off or put on a bathing suit.

Now, look at where you are kicking ass in life. Dig in and find the why and the habits that make it happen.

Now apply it to your health.

48. How Much Time do You Waste?

How much time do you waste? Too much? Me too!

I don't have time to work out.

I can't eat healthily, it's too hard.

I hear this all the time.

In the next sentence, I can ask the same person about four hundred Netflix shows, and they have seen them all.

We all lie to ourselves about this. I have two simple solutions for you.

1. The first thing you should do is get a notebook and start tracking your day. Write down everything you do and what time. Don't think about anything, when you do something, write it down. Do this for three days.

2. The second thing you do is identify the time-wasters. I guarantee the biggest one right now is your phone and social media.

Now fill the gaps with the things you could do to feel great and look awesome.

Time is the one thing you can NEVER get back. Track it and maximize your life.

49. Back to the Basics

I find it funny, but I repeat myself a lot these days. What about? The basics. Why? There are many reasons so let's dive in.

The first and probably most important is that the basics are what builds the foundation for you to make improvements.

It's as simple as the house with no foundation analogy, obviously the house caves in on itself with no foundation.

It is the same for working out and health. If you are getting only four to five hours a sleep a night and then try and go "kill it" in the gym, it's a recipe for disaster. In this case sleep is the foundation.

If I had to pin it down to exactly what the basics are, it would be below and in this order:

- Sleep
- Hydration
- Stress reduction

- Whole foods-based diet
- Strength training
- Moving daily (10,000 steps or similar)

Do you know how many people skip this but do a one-hour boot camp and wonder why they are still fat, sick and tired?

There are nuances to each one of these and need some context, but for now you get the point.

I get it, the basics aren't sexy and can be tedious, but I hate to break it to you, that's how you reach any goal you set.

50. Conclusion

It's not a coincidence I wrapped up with the basics. I cannot, let me repeat, cannot stress the importance of the basics when it comes to anything you want to be good at in life. If there was only one thing you got out of this book was the fact the without your health you have nothing then I am happy. Job complete.

Being a high performer in life requires you to do the little things day in and day out, and that requires daily discipline.

I hope you can find the discipline to make health a top priority so you can kick ass in life for a very long time.

If you would like to find out more information on my programs, please check me out here:

Website: www.damonmoschetto.com

Facebook - https://www.facebook.com/damon.moschetto/

Instagram - https://www.instagram.com/damonmoschetto/